YOUR KNOWLEDGE HAS VALUE

AF135546

- We will publish your bachelor's and master's thesis, essays and papers

- Your own eBook and book - sold worldwide in all relevant shops

- Earn money with each sale

Upload your text at www.GRIN.com and publish for free

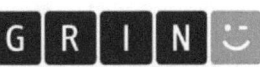

Bibliographic information published by the German National Library:

The German National Library lists this publication in the National Bibliography; detailed bibliographic data are available on the Internet at http://dnb.dnb.de .

Imprint:

Copyright © 2019 GRIN Verlag
Print and binding: Books on Demand GmbH, Norderstedt Germany
ISBN: 9783346103581

This book at GRIN:

https://www.grin.com/document/512610

Gizaw Mekonnen

Review on Impact of Mycotoxin Contamination on Animal Health and Productivity

GRIN Verlag

GRIN - Your knowledge has value

Since its foundation in 1998, GRIN has specialized in publishing academic texts by students, college teachers and other academics as e-book and printed book. The website www.grin.com is an ideal platform for presenting term papers, final papers, scientific essays, dissertations and specialist books.

Visit us on the internet:

http://www.grin.com/

http://www.facebook.com/grincom

http://www.twitter.com/grin_com

REVEIW ON IMPACT OF MYCOTOXIN CONTAMINATION ON ANIMAL HEALTH AND PRODUCTIVITY

PREPARED BY

GIZAW MEKONNEN

SENIOR SEMINAR PAPER SUBMITTED TO SCHOOL OF VETERINARY MEDICINE, WOLAITA SODO UNIVERSITY, SENIOR SEMINAR COURSE ON ANIMAL HEALTH (VETM 522)

MARCH, 2019
WOLAITA SODO, ETHIOPIA

ACKNOWLEDGEMENTS

First of all I would like to thanks my God. Without his blessing this senior seminar presentation would not have been successfully. Next to this I would like to give regards and thanks to my advisor Dr. Gishu Beriso to providing me with her knowledge and understandings. I would like to thank University of W S U, Faculty of Veterinary Medicine for the providing to us to do this seminar presentation and all academic staff as well as computer lab technician. I would also be great full to announce thanks to my families by helping different materials and my wife Aynalem Kensiro.

Table of Contents   page

LIST OF TABLES Pages

LIST OF FIGURES

Page

LIST OF ABBREVIATION

ZEA	Zearalenone
AFs	Aflatoxins
OTA	Ochratoxin A
F	fumonisins
DAS	Diaeetoxyscirpenol
UGT	uridine 5'-diphosphate glucuronosyltransferase
3α-HSD	3α -hydroxysteroid dehydrogenase
3β –HSD	3β–hydroxysteroid dehydrogenase
DNA	Deoxyribonucleic acid

SUMMARY

Mycotoxins are secondary metabolism of filamentous fungi, which under suitable temperature and humidity conditions, and found in various foods and feeds, causing negative effect for human and animal health. There are different mycotoxins which have agricultural and economic importance including aflatoxins, ochratoxins, trichothecenes, zearalenone, fumonisins, tremorgenic toxins, and ergot alkaloids. Mycotoxins occur more frequently in areas with a hot and humid climate, favourable for the growth of molds, they can also be found in temperate zones. In comparison to monogastric species, ruminant animals are generally less susceptible to the adverse effects caused by contamination of feeds with mycotoxins because presence of rumen microflora in rumen. However, a number of mycotoxins resist rumen degradation, causing distinct clinical signs of intoxication. Dairy cattle can be exposed to different number of mycotoxins because complex feeding diet originating from different feed materials such as roughage and concentrates. Exposure of diary catte to these mycotoxins may result in unexpected health problem. Due to apre-existing negative energy balance, cows in the transition period are considered to be particularly sensitive to the exposure to feeds. The variation of mycotoxin occurence due to different factors, including agricultural practices and climatic conditions .Aflatoxins (AFs)are found in maize and peanuts, aswell as in tree nuts and dried fruits. OTA is found mainly in cereals, but significant levels of contamination may also occur in wine, coffee, spices and dried fruits. Other products of concern are beans, roasted coffee and cocoa, malt and beer, bread and bakery products, wines and grape juices, spices, poultry meat and kidneys, pig kidneys and pork sausages. The production of secondary metabolism is the effect of Fungal metabolism. Secondary metabolites, are formed from a relatively small number of branch points of primary metabolic pathways. Among them some of these secondary metabolites are used as antibiotics, while others are very toxic and carcinogenic to humans and animals. Economic impact associated with mycotoxicosis including: Slower growth rates, Poor conception rates, inconsistent manure, Increased disease susceptibility, Reduced production performance, loss of animal and human life, veterinary and public cost of treatment.

Key word: *Diary cattle, Mongastric species, Mycotoxin, Ruminant.*

1. INTRODUCTION

Mycotoxins are toxins produced by fungi which can contaminate food crop, or entire food crops, throughout the food chain. These mycotoxins have some effects in animals and humans including effect on agricultural productivity, toxic effect in animals and negative effect on immune system that lead decline defense mechanism as well as low growth rate.The toxic effects of these metabolites in mammals (including humans) is known as mycotoxicosis(Kaushik,2013).

Mycotoxins are a structurally diverse group of mostly small molecular weight compounds, produced mainly by the secondary metabolism of some filamentous fungi, or molds, which under suitable temperature and humidity conditions, and may develop on various foods and feeds, causing serious risks for human and animal health. Mycotoxins are secondary metabolites that have no biochemical significance in fungal growth and development; however, they vary from simple C4 compounds, e.g.,moniliformin, to complex substances such as the phomopsins(Dinis*et al.*, 2007).

There are different types of mycotoxins which have agro-economic signifinance and public health cocern including aflatoxins (AF), ochratoxins (OT), trichothecenes, zearalenone (ZEN), fumonisins (F), tremorgenic toxins, and ergot alkaloids. These toxins account for millions of dollars annually in losses worldwide in human health, animal health, and condemned agricultural products (Zain.M.E., 2011)

The production of mycotoxins and fungal multiplication depend on environmental factors, moisture content, humidity,temperatures especially during tropical conditions (Mohd R., *et al.,*2013).The processing such as poor harvesting practices, improper storage and less than optimal conditions during transportation, processing, and marketing can contribute to the growth of fungi and increase the risk of the major food spoilage agent caused by mycotoxin production (Khazaeli *et al.,*2014)

Depending on environmental conditions like storage, time of harvesting and climate conditions as well as way of harvesting, different fungi colonize their host and produce mycotoxins. Some of these toxins trigger immune deficiency, lower production in livestock and are carcinogenic.

mycotoxins are resistant against treatments during food processing because of that reason once contaminated, mycotoxins containing feed and foods are condemned (Kagot V. *et al.,2019.)*

Mycotoxins impact in animal production includes the reduced productivity of animals, the increased cost of health and veterinary care, disposal of contaminated feeds, and investment in research and applications to reduce severity of the mycotoxin problem (Denli M., 2015).

Therefore, the objective of this seminar paper is

> ➢ To review the frequency and degree of occurrence of mycotoxins in different feedstuffs
> ➢ To review toxicological effects of mycotoxin intake on the performance of the main livestock (*i.e.*, poultry, swine, cattle, goats and sheep)
> ➢ To understand effect of mycotoxin on animals and its economic impacts.

2. LITERATURE REVIEW

2.1. occurrence and signifinance of mycotoxins

Mycotoxicoses are diseases produced from most common fungi toxinknown as Mycotoxins directly or in combination with other primary stressors such as pathogens (Raju and Devegowda, 2000). Mycotoxicoses in humans or animals are characterized as food or feed related, non-contagious, non-transferable, non-infectious, and non-traceable to microorganisms other than fungi. Clinical symptoms usually subside upon removal of contaminated food or feed. A wide range of commodities can be contaminated with mycotoxins both pre- and post-harvest (CAST, 2003).

The occurrence of the fungi in the field is related to several factors, including agricultural practices and climatic conditions .There are different fungi species , such as *Aspergillus fumigatus*, *Penicillium roqueforti*, *P. paneum*, *F. oxysporum* and *Monascus ruber* that are able to tolerate both high levels of organic acids and carbon dioxide in addition to low availability of oxygen . In particular, presence of oxygen in some parts of silage during storage or oxygen penetration during feed-out and aerobic spoilage phases could allow mold growth and mycotoxin production. In high quality silage, lactic acid bacteria are effective in hindering any mold growth, but just a small raise in the oxygen concentration could provide the right growth conditions for fungi such as *P. roqueforti* and *P. paneum*. Indeed, if most of acetic and lactic acids as well as carbon dioxide evaporate and more oxygen is present, nearly all cereal-associated filamentous fungi may grow.The variation of mycotoxin occurence and concentration depend on environment related factors (Gallo A.,2015).

Aflatoxins (AFTs) are found in maize and peanuts, as well as in tree nuts and dried fruits. OTA is found mainly in cereals, but significant levels of contamination may also occur in wine, coffee, spices and dried fruits. Other products of concern are beans, roasted coffee and cocoa, malt and beer, bread and bakery products, wines and grape juices, spices, poultry meat and kidneys, pig kidneys and pork sausages (Milicevic *et al.,* 2008).

Table 1 Some mycotoxins, their sources and potential toxicities source (Suttajit M,2019)

Toxins	Producing fungi	Toxicities
Aflatoxin	*Aspergillus flavus*	Hepatocarcinogen
	Aspergillus parasiticus	and fatty liver
Citreoviridin	*Penicillium viridicatum*	Cardiac beri-beri
Citrinin	*Penicillium vindicatum*	Nephrotoxin
	Penicillium citrinum	
Cyclochlorotine	*Penicillium islandicum*	Hepatotoxin
Cytochalasin E	*Aspergillus clavatus*	Cytotoxicity
Maltoryzine	*Aspergillus oryzae*	
Ochratoxins	*Aspergillus ochraceus*	Hepatotoxin
Patulin	*Penicillium c-expansum*	Brain & lung hemorrhage
	Penicillium patulum	and carcinogenicity
PR Toxin	*Penicillium requeforti*	
Rubratoxin	*Penicillium rubrum*	Liver hemmorrhage and fatty infiltration
Rugulosin	*Penicillium islandicum*	Nephrosis& liver damage
Sterigmatocystin	*Aspergillus flavus*	Hepatocarcinogen
	Aspergillusversicolor	
Tremorgens	*Penicillium and Aspergillus*	
Trichothecenes	*Fusarium graminearum*	Cytotoxicity
Vomitoxin (Deoxynivalenol)	*Fusarium graminearum*	Vomiting
Zearalenone	*Fusarium*	Hyper-estrogenic effect

2.2.   Aflatoxin

AFs are difuranocoumarin derivatives produced by a polyketide pathway by many strains of A. flavus and A. parasiticus; in particular, A. flavus is a common contaminant in agriculture. Aspergillus bombycis, Aspergillus ochraceoroseus, Aspergillus nomius, and Aspergillus pseudotamari are also aflatoxin-producing species, but they are encountered less frequently (Peterson *et al.*, 2001). Aflatoxins are found occasionally in milk, cheese, peanuts, cottonseed , nuts, almonds, figs, spices, and a variety of other foods and feeds. Milk, eggs, and meat products are sometimes contaminated because of the animal consumption of aflatoxin contaminated feed. Cottonseed, Brazil nuts, copra, various tree nuts and pistachio nuts are the other commodities quite susceptible to the invasion of aflatoxin producing fungi.

Figures 1 contaminated corn by aflatoxin

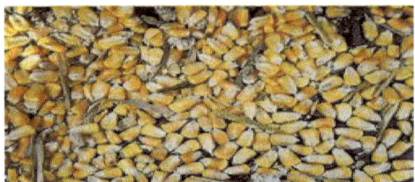

Source(https://tse4.mm.bing.net/th?id=OIP.IC6jATwlp48pjFoKfUnwFQHaE6&pid=15.1&P=0 &w=252&h=168) on 12/3/2019

Aflatoxin contamination has been linked to increased mortality in farm animals and thus significantly lowers the value of grains as an animal feed and as an export commodity. Milk products can also serve as an indirect source of aflatoxin. When cows consume aflatoxin-contaminated feeds, they metabolically biotransform aflatoxin B1 into a hydroxylated form called aflatoxin M1 (Van Egmond, 1989).

Aflatoxins cause damage in liver including cancer, decreased milk and egg production, and suppression of immunity in animals consuming low dietary concentrations. While the young are most susceptible, all ages are affected; clinical signs include GI dysfunction, decreased reproductivity, decreased feed utilization and efficiency, anemia, and jaundice. Nursing animals may be affected by exposure to aflatoxin metabolites secreted in the milk (CAST.,2003).

Acute aflatoxicosis induced abdominal pain, vomiting, edema, and death .In addition to that there are other reported clinical signs of acute aflatoxicosis in mammals include inappetence, lethargy, ataxia, rough hair coat, and pale, enlarged fatty livers whereas Symptoms of chronic aflatoxicosis include reduced feed efficiency and milk production, jaundice, and decreased appetite. Aflatoxin lowers resistance to diseases and interferes with vaccine-induced immunity (Mohd-Redzwan et al., 2013).

2.3. Ochratoxin

Ochratoxins are closely related derivatives of isocoumarin, linked to an amino acid, L-β-phenylalanine. Among nine types of ochratoxins, ochratoxin A is the most effective one. Ochratoxins are produced in maize, peanuts, beans etc(Neleesh,2019) The major species implicated in OTA production includes Aspergillus ochraceus, Aspergillus carbonarius, Aspergillus melleus, Aspergillus sclerotiorum, Aspergillus sulphureus, Pichia verrucossum. However, Aspergillus niger and Pichia purpurescens are less important OTA producers (Benford et al., 2001).

Ochratoxinsare secondary metabolites synthesized mainly by *Aspergillus* and *Penicillium* that contaminate agricultural products and have negative effects on animals and humans.There are different toxic effect of OTA in animal cells including the inhibition of protein synthesis, lipid peroxidation, DNA damage and oxidoreductive stress .However,blocking of protein synthesis is most common toxic effect. OTA has the mutagenic effects in mammals due to DNA damage induction.In addition OTA has genotoxic carcinogen role of OTA, due to the induction of oxidative DNA lesions(Battacone G. et al.,2010)

Ochratoxin A (OTA) is mycotoxins that have public health importance.The presence of OTA in animal feed depend on the direct and indirect fungal contamination of animal products.OTA formation occurs mainly after harvesting on insufficiently dried cereal and cereal products. The formation of OTA depend on several factors including environmental conditions, such as temperature and water activity as well as the type and integrity of the seeds. While *A.*

*ochraceus*grows better in oilseeds (peanuts and soybeans) than in grain crops, such as wheat and corn, *P. verrucosum* may grow better in wheat and corn(Denli M.and Perez Jose F.,2010).

The detoxification potential of ruminants and the generally low indication for OTA occurrence in forages, it is not surprising that OTA contamination is not at the centre of mycotoxin concerns in ruminant feeds. However, some OTA contamination of diets cannot be excluded given the variety of feeds offered to ruminants. While it can sometimes occur at concentrations high enough to cause major losses in health and performance of monogastrics, a more likely scenario for ruminants is to find a lower level of OTA occurrence in diets and only subclinical disorders related with OTA (Mobashar M., 2010).

2.4. Zearalenone

Zearalenone (ZEA), one of the mycotoxins, mainly comes from the feed which was contaminated by some Fusarium and Gibberella species in the field and farm or in the period and storage. Although before harvest time, the cereals infected by Fusarium may accumulate ZEA in the field, numerous evidence has revealed that high level of ZEA could be naturally occurring in the corn-based animal feeds, and thus be attributed to the improper storage methods rather than occurring in the field. The trade of these contaminated cereal commodities may contribute to the worldwide dispersal of ZEA. Several studies have shown that ZEA exerted different mechanisms of toxicity in different cell types at different doses. ZEA and its derivatives can not only stimulate the cell growth but also inhibit the cell viability and cause cell death including apoptosis and necrosi s(Zheng W. *et al.*, 2010).

Zearalenone (ZEA) is a phenolic resorcyclic acid lactone produced primarily by Fusarium,and is with potent oestrogenic properties and oestrogen effect in common animals like cattle sheep, pigs as well as wheat,corn,oats and sorghum as substrates of ZEA (Schwarzer, 2009). Zearalenone (ZEA), one of the mycotoxins, mainly comes from the feed which was contaminated by some Fusarium and Gibberella species in the field and farm or in the period and storage as well as it is bind with estrogen receptors and compete with 17 estradiol (Chang,H,*et al.*, 2017).

The main way for human and animals exposure to ZEA is consuming the cereal grains and derived products which may be contaminated by toxigenic fungi species of Fusarium in field or during food production, processing and storage(Ismaiel, A.A. *et al.*,2015). These toxigenic fungi are considered as significantly harmful pathogens due to producing mycotoxin in the safety and quality of cereal grains (Ren, G.X.;*et al.*,2018). ZEA has the carcinogenic effect because of stimulating the cells proliferation. ZEA could promote cells proliferation and also promote cell migration and colony formation which are the center reason of carcinogenic property (Abassi, H.; *et al.*,2016).

ZEA is a non-steroidal estrogenic mycotoxin that is implicated in the reproductive disorders of farm animals and hyperoestrogenic syndromes in humans (Kotowicz *et al.*, 2014). Toxicological studies of ZEA revealed its effects on the reproductive system, including enlargment of uterus, altered reproductive organs(ovaries,uterus,oviduct ,vagina and others, fertility problems, as well as abnormal level of progesterone and estradiol. Besides, the ingestion of ZEA during pregnancy reduced fetal weight and survival rate of embryo (Zhang *et al.*, 2014).

3. NEGATIVE EFFECTS OF MYCOTOXINS ON NON- RUMINANTS

3.1 Poultry

Mycotoxins have serious health problem on livestock animals. In poultry production alone, mycotoxins have been linked to mouth lesions, yellow livers, gizzard erosions and poor gut integrity. Many of the world's biggest poultry integrators pay very close attention to their grain and feed quality because of the effects these challenges may have on poultry health and on profit margins. When it comes to organic poultry production, however, the more stringent regulations also present unique challenges (Reyes M: 2019).

Mcotoxins are commonly affected all poultry species. The response of poultry species to mycotoxin challenges vary, but clinical signs of mycotoxicosis can be difficult to detect. Careful monitoring, recognitions of symptoms, and postmortem diagnosis merge with adequate feed analyses are most accurate mean of mycotoxicosis diagnosis within large flocks of poultry (http://www.knowmycotoxins.com/species/poultry).

In poultry, ducks are the most sensitive to aflatoxins, followed by turkey, broiler and layers. Duration of exposure, as well as age, is as important as the level of aflatoxins in feed. The following symptoms have smaller eggs and reduced eggshell quality, coccidiosis, vaccine failure, reduced immunity, lower resistance to diseases, bacteria, viruses and of course reduced performance (Iheshiulor et al., 2011)

The aflatoxicosis in poultry can b e characterized by different effects including hepatic dysfuction,liverfat,poor feed effeciency,changes in organ weights, reduction in serum protein levels, carcass bruising, poor pigmentation(carcasses, egg ,yolk), enzymes inactivation lead problem in digestion of starch, protien, lipids and nucleic acids whereas ochratoxin toxicity in poultry cause weakness, anemia, reduced growth rate and egg production, poor excessive mortality at high dietary concentrations(G. R. Murugesan et al., 2015)

The synerstic interaction of AF and OTA are co-contaminants of poultry feed. OTA prevents the major effects of AF (i.e., fatty, yellow, enlarged and friable liver). kindey is most common target organ in this synergistic effect of interaction. In addition to that OTA reduces the ability to diagnose aflatoxicosis in the field . The combination of AF and T2 toxin is the same as the interaction between AF and OTA, and exhibit synergistic toxicity. In acute mycotoxicosis, ingestion of high level of mycotoxins lead to death of poultry and reduce productivity (G. R. Murugesan *et al.*, 2015).

3.2. Pigs

Pigs are very sensitive to mycotoxins. The factors that determine the levels to which animals are affected. These factors are age of pigs,phase of production in pigs and concentration of mycotoxins in feed.However,mycotoxin contamination at minnium levels reduce performance in pigs,affect immune system of pigs and health status and cause deaths.Mycotoxins are mainly affect young pigs and breeding sows/boars (http://www.knowmycotoxins.com/species/pigs)

The mycotoxins have different negative effects on reproduction.Zearalenone, ergot alkaloids and trichothecenes are common cause fertility problem in pigs.howeverzearalenone is most common mycotoxins among causes of reproductive mycotoxicoses .Reproductive failure and a drop in reproductive performances brought on by mycotoxins can be defined as reproductive mycotoxicoses. The influence of zearalenone on litter size due to negative impact on fertilization, but also by embryonic and fetal death of the piglets.due to the negative impact on the luteinizing effect (A.kanoral, D. Maes.,2009)

The conversion of ZEA to α-ZOL in the liver, the small intestines, and even in granulose cells and the low glucuronidation capacity in most pig breeds are important factor for the high sensitivity of pigs towards the endocrine effects of ZEA (keller L.,2015)

The different mycotoxins combined together can affect immunity system of pigs. The mycotoxin found in feed of pregnant sows cause embryonic and fetal death. Feeding lactating sows with grains naturally contaminated with Fusariummycotoxins results in reduced feed intake and increased body weight loss in piglets, but no changes in milk composition or milk production are detected. The reduced feed intake and losses of body tissues tend to increase the weaning to estrus interval (Radulovic.J.Z.P., 2013)

3.3. Horses

The contamination of pasture, mouldy conserved forage, purchased feeds and bedding by mycotoxins cause serious the health problem of equine animals.many horses are high value animals with a much longer life span than agricultural livestock because of their status in human society. Athletic horses and horses need to competitions means a higher level of stress as a result of travelling and competing. This can have a negative effect on the immune system, which means horses can be particularly susceptible to mycotoxins (http: // www. Know mycotoxins .com / species / equine).

The commonly mycotoxin in equine are the toxins produced by Fusarium moniliforme which cause equine leukoencephalomalacia and acute neurotoxicity. These diseases were attributed to consumption of corn contaminated with FB1 and moniliformin toxins. Clinical manifestation of equine leukoencephalomalacia include ataxia, paresis, apathy hypersensitivity, impaired locomotor function, necrosis of cerebral white matter, and lesions in the cerebral cortex. Bean-hulls poisoning is another mycotoxin-related disease that has been known in Hokkaido (Japan) for seven decades because of the availability of bean-hulls as a cheap source of feed and bedding for horses. Clinical symptoms include central nervous system dysfunction, rapid heartbeat, diminished ocular reflexes, and death (Zain M. E.2011).

4. NEGATIVE EFFECTS OF MYCOTOXINS ON RUMINANTS

Ruminants such as cattle, sheep, goats and deer are less known for their sensitivity to the negative effects of mycotoxins than are non-ruminants. However, production (milk, beef, or wool), reproduction and growth can be altered when ruminants consume mycotoxin-contaminated feed for extended periods of time. Beef and dairy cattle, sheep, goats and deer are among ruminants that have been investigated. Acute aflatoxicosis in cattle has been thoroughly described. Clinical signs consist of reduced feed consumption, dramatic drops in milk production, weight loss, liver damage and reduced immune system function and rumen metabolism in cattle. Increasing AF in cattle feed to levels such as 10, 26, 56.4, 81.1 and 108.5 µg kg^{-1} has been shown to significantly reduce feed intake at each level in a dose-dependent manner(Iheshiulor*et al.*,2011) .

4.1. Cattle

Bovine Mycotoxicosis in cattle cause decreased values in serum total protein, albumin, alpha globulin, beta globulin, and gamma globulin. Decrease in serum globulin in mycotoxicated animals might be due to the adverse effect of mycotox-ins on synthesis of total proteins and globulin. Mycotoxins cause inhibition of DNA and protein synthesis as well as immunosup-pression due to the inflammation and cirrhosis of liver and kidneys.(Hassan *et al.*,2012).

Aflatoxins have negatively effect production, immune system function, and rumen metabolism in cattle. However Ochratoxins have toxic effect to cattle when fed alone in naturally occurring doses. Barley naturally-contaminated with OTA (390–540 lg/kg) and low levels of AFB1 (12–13 lg/kg) did not induce any significant clinical symptoms in 12-week-old calves. The absence of a toxic effect may have been due to the ruminal microbial degradation and detoxification AFB1 has potential to inhibit bovine lymphocyte blastogenesis (Zain Mohamed E.,2011)

Table 2. Major toxigenic fungi and the mycotoxins thought to be the most prevalent and potentially toxic to dairy cattle

Fungal genera	Mycotoxin
Aspergillus	Aflatoxin, Ochratoxin, Sterigmatocytsin, Fumitremorgens, FumitoxinsCyclopiazonoic Acid, GliotoxinFumigaclavines
	Deoxynivalenol, Zearalenone, T-2 Toxin, Fumonisin, Moniliformin, Nivalenol, Diacetoxyscirpenol, Butenolide, Neosolaniol, Fusaric Acid, Fusarochromanone, Wortmannin, Fusarin C, Fusaproliferin
Penicillium	Ochratoxin, PR Toxin, Patulin, Penicillic Acid, Citrinin, Penetrem, Cyclopiazonic Acid, Roquefortine, Isofumigaclavines A and B, Mycophenolic Acid
Claviceps	Ergot alkaloids in seed/grain of small grains, sorghum, grasses
Epichloe and Neotyphodium	Ergo alkaloids in fescue grass
Stachybotrys	Stachybotryotoxins, trichothecenes

Source (Lon W.W.,andWintson M.Hagler,Jr.,2005)

4.2. Sheep

Sheep are the most resistant species to mycotoxicosis than cattle and sheep .In sheep especially,lambs fed AF at 2.5 mg/kg of feed daily for 21 days show clinical aflatoxicosis including hepatic and nephritic lesions, altered mineral metabolism, and increased size and weight of the liver and kidney. The mineral deficiencies due to aflatoxicosis were leads to lower feed intake and to the liver and kidney malfunctions as a result of AF intoxication. .(Zain Mohamed E.2011).

Lambs are commonly affected by AFs. Lambs affected by aflatoxicosis show clinical manifestation including decrease production performance,abnormality of liver with lesion and even death. Diaeetoxyscirpenol (DAS) is a trichothecenemycotoxin . Like T-2 toxin, DAS has been described as radiomimetic with regard to lymphoid tissues and gastrointestinal epithelium, as a contact necrotizing agent for lingual and buccal mucosa, and an inhibitor of DNA and protein synthesis (Harvey R. B. 1995).

4.3. Other Ruminants

Except cattle and sheep, ruminants have variable resistance to mycotoxins. In weanling goats ,Levels of AF at 95 mg/kg of feed had no effects on body weight gain and clinical signs cannot detect of aflatoxicosis. However,Signs of toxic effects were only detected through serum profile and sphingolipid analysis. In a study with white-tailed deer fawn fed 800 mg/kg AF over an 8-week-period, acute injuries in the liver were indicated by increased serum bile acid concentrations and hepatic lesions Impact of mycotoxins on humans and animals (Zain Mohamed E.2011).

5. METABOLISM OF MYCOTOXINS

The challenges of mycotoxin metabolism, determining the factors that influence the extent of mycotoxin contamination of food, and devising new methods of reducing or eliminating their contamination of food has become an important aspect of clinical and environmental mycology. The production of secondary metabolism is the effect of Fungal metabolism Secondary metabolites, are formed from a relatively small number of branch points of primary metabolic pathways. Among them some of these secondary metabolites are used as antibiotics, while others are very toxic and carcinogenic to humans and animals (Anyanwu.E.C. *et al.*, 2004).

ZEA is commonly metabolism in the liver and intestine. It was transformed into α-zearalenol (α-ZEA), β-zearalenol (β-ZEA), zearalanone (ZAN), α-zearalanol (α-ZAL) and β-zearalanol (β-ZAL) and all of which were subsequently conjugated to glucuronic acid .There are two way of metabolism including Phase-I and phase-II. At the phase-I, the ketone group in ZEA or ZAN which is a semi-synthetic mycoestrogen and a derivative of ZEA was reduced by aliphatic hydroxylation to metabolize the corresponding alcohol. ZEA was converted to α-ZEL and β-ZEL and ZAN was converted to α-ZAL and β-ZAL, which was catalyzed by 3α -hydroxysteroid dehydrogenase (3α-HSD) or 3β–hydroxysteroid dehydrogenase (3β -HSD) . At the phase- II the metabolites from phase-I were glucuronidated and sulfated. The glucuronic acid group was supplied by uridine 5′-diphosphate glucuronic acid (UDPGA) which was catalyzed by uridine 5′-diphosphate glucuronosyltransferase (UGT) (Zheng W. *et al.*,2010).

Metabolism of AFB1 involves oxidative reactions by members of the cYP450 supergene family of isoenzymes. Different cYP450 isoenzymes result in AFB1 metabolites of varying carcinogenic potential. There are four way of metabolism of AFB1 include O-dealkylation to AFP1, ketoreduction to AFL, epoxidation to AFB1-8,9-epoxide, and hydroxylation to AFM, AFP1, AFQ1, or AFB2a.In first phase ofaflatoxin metabolism converts original molecules into more hydrophilic compounds utilizing mainly enzymatic hydrolytic and oxidative–reduction reactions.In Phase II, react origi-nal molecule or its metabolites with nucleophilic molecules such as glutathione, glucuronides, and sulfonides (Dohnal.V*et al.*,2014). Aflatoxin B1 is metabolized by microsomal enzymes to different metabolites through hydroxylation, hydration, demethylation and epoxidation in liver . Aflatoxicol is the only metabolite of AFB1 produced by a soluble cytoplasmic reductase enzyme system in liver. As a result, metabolism of proteins, carbohydrates and lipids in liver is seriously impaired by AFB1. The toxin inhibits RNA polymerase and subsequent protein synthesis at a faster rate in ducks than in rats probably because of faster liver metabolism of AFB1 in ducks than in rats (Dhanasekaran D.*et al.*,2015)

After oral consumption of OTA-contaminated feed,absorption of OTA absorption in the blood via the gastrointestinal tract slow elimination in urine and feces The disease caused by OTA exposure is known as *ochratoxicosis*, and the primary target is the kidney (Denli M.,2015).

6. ECONOMIC IMPACT OF MYCOTOXINS

Mycotoxins have significant economic and commercial impact, in that both the productivity and nutritive value of the infected cereal and forage is affected. There are different consideration for observation and evaluation of the economic impact of mycotoxins on animals and on humans. However, some criteria include reduce amount of a crop in market, reduced value of contaminated products in domestic markets, regulatory rejection of products by high-value markets, and damages suffered via afflicted livestock, including disease, morbidity, mortality, and contamination of animal products as well as loss of livestock production and veterinary cost (Iheshiulor *et al.*,2011).

The economic impact of mycotoxins on animals and humans are on a single aspect of mycotoxin exposure or contamination because of that Formulas for worldwide economic impact have been difficult to develop (Hussein and Brasel, 2001)..

Mycotoxins have economic impacts in numerous crops, especially wheat, maize, peanuts and other nut crops, cottonseed, and coffee. The Food and Agriculture Organization has estimated that 25% of the world's crops are affected by mycotoxins each year, with annual losses of around 1 billion metric tons of foods and food products. Economic losses including yield loss due to diseases induced by toxigenic fungi, reduced crop value resulting from mycotoxin contamination, losses in animal productivity; and human health costs. Other economic loss in case additional cost such as the cost of management at all levels– prevention, sampling, mitigation, litigation, and research costs. These economic impacts are felt all along the food and feed supply chains: crop producers, animal producers, grain handlers and distributors, processors, consumers, and society as a whole (due to health careimpactsand productivity losses (https://www.apsnet.org/edcenter/intropp/topics/Mycotoxins/Pages/EconomicImpact.aspx) on 13/3/2019 In animals, AFs can be considered as a cause of economic losses due to lower resistance to diseases, counteraction of vaccine-induced immunity, and adverse effects on growth and reproduction (CAST, 2003).

7. CONCLUSION AND RECOMMENDATION

Mycotoxins are poisonous chemical compounds produced by kingdom fungi. There are five mycotoxins in animal feed including :deoxynivalenol/Nivalenol, zearalenone, ochratoxin, fumonisins and aflatoxins. Apart from practicing good sanitary measures, awareness has to be created to indicate the toxic effects associated with mycotoxin poisonings in humans and livestock. Now the day, there are wide gaps still exist on the toxicological effects of feeding animals mycotoxin-contaminated feeds. The toxicity of many of the compounds is high so that natural contamination of foods produces the threat of possible carcinogenesis and natural contamination of livestock feeds produces death losses or a severe reduction or both in livestock productivity. Incidences of mycotoxicoses in livestock are usually characterized by a rapid onset with sudden death losses. Mycotoxicosis have Economic impact including: Slower growth rates, Poor conception rates, inconsistent manure, Increased disease susceptibility, Reduced production performance, loss of animal and human life, veterinary and public cost of treatment..The risk of exposure to the occurrence of mycotoxin poisoning in livestock production could be reduced by recognizing the field conditions and farm storage conditions under which these molds develop.In general mycotoxins have negative effects on animals and humans.

Based on above conclusion,following recommendation are forwarded

➢ The good sanitary measures should be taken to reduce incidence of mycotoxicosis which cause by mycotoxins.

➢ Owners or farmers should aware about mycotoxins and its impact and sources.

➢ Mycotoxins levels regulation should be implemented in countries.

➢ Additional current preventive measures with the use of agents that are bind toxins,thus limiting their bioavailability in animals.

➢ The development of physical, chemical and biotechnological tools to improve seed production, cultivation, harvest and storage of forages and cereals, is essential to reduce the level of contamination of foods and feeds.

8. REFERENCES

A.Kanora1 , D. Maes(2009) The role of mycotoxins in pig reproduction Veterinarni Medicina, 54, 12: 565–576

A.M.P. Dinis, C.M. Lino, A.S. (2007)PenaOchratoxin A in nephropathic patients from two cities of central zone in Portugal *J. Pharmaceut. Biomed. Anal.*, **44** , pp. 553–557

Abassi, H.; Ayed-Boussema, I.; Shirley, S.; Abid, S.; Bacha, H.; Micheau, O.(2016)The mycotoxinzearalenone enhances cell proliferation,colony formation and promotes cell migrationin the human colon carcinoma cell line HCT116. *Toxicol.Lett.***254**, 1–7.

Anyanwu E. C., Morad M., and Campbell Andrew W.,(2004) . Metabolism of Mycotoxins, Intracellular Functions of Vitamin B12, and Neurological Manifestations in Patients with Chronic Toxigenic Mold Exposures *The Scientific World Journal* **4,** 736–745

BattaconeG.,AnnaNuddaA.,andPulina G.,(2010)   Effects of Ochratoxin A on Livestock Production.*Toxins,***2,**1796-1824

Benford, D., Boyle, C., Dekant, W., Fuchs, E., Gaylor, D.W., Hard, G., McGregory, D.B., Pitt, J.I., Plestina, R., Shephard, G., Solfrizzo, M., Verger, P.J.P., Walker, R., 2001.Ochratoxin A Safety Evaluation of Certain Mycotoxins in Food.WHO Food Additives Series 47.FAO Food and Nutrition Paper, vol. 74. WHO Geneva, Switzerland, pp. 281–415.

CAST,(2003). Mycotoxins: Risks in Plant, Animal and Human Systems. Report No. 139. *Council for Agricultural Science and Technology,* Ames, Iowa, USA

Chang,H.;Kim,W.;Park,J.H.;Kim,D.;Kim,C.R.;Chung,S.;Lee,C.(2017)Theoccurrenceofzearalen oneinSouth Korean feedstuffs between 2009 and 2016. *Toxins,***9**

Denli M.(2015).implications of mycotoxins in livestock feeds.*AgroLife Scientific Journal*, 4, 1, 2015

DenliM.,Perez Jose F.,(2010) Ochratoxins in Feed, a Risk for Animal and Human Health: Control Strategies. *Toxins* **2**(5),1065-1077

Dhanasekaran D., Shanmugapriya S., ThajuddinN.,andPanneerselvam A. (2015).Aflatoxins and Aflatoxicosis in Human and Animals. *Aflatoxins –Biochemistry and Molecular Biology* 222-254

DohnalVlastimil ,WuQinghua ,KucaKamil(2014) Metabolism of aflatoxins: key enzymes and interindividual as well as interspecies differences. *Archives of Toxicology* **88**:1635–1644

G. R. Murugesan,D. R. Ledoux,K. Naehrer,F. Berthiller,T. J. Applegate,B. Grenier,T. D. Phillips, G. Schatzmay(2015) Prevalence and effects of mycotoxins on poultry health and performance, andrecent development in mycotoxin counteracting strategies.*Poultry Science.***94** 6 1298–1315.

Gallo A., Giuberti G., FrisvadJens C., TerenzioBertuzzi T., NielsenKristian F.,(2015) Review on Mycotoxin Issues in Ruminants: Occurrence in Forages, Effects of Mycotoxin Ingestion on Health Status and Animal Performance and Practical Strategies to Counteract Their Negative Effects. *Toxins* 7, 3057-3111

Harvey R. B. ,EdringtonT. S., Kubena L. F., ElissaldeM. H., Corrier D. E., Rottinghaus G. E.,(1995).Effect of Aflatoxin and Diacetoxyscirpenol in Ewe Lambs.Bull. Environ. Contam.Toxicol.**54**,325-330

Hassan, A.A.; Howayda, M. El Shafei; Noha, H. Oraby; Rasha, M.H. Sayed El Ahl and Mogeda, K. Mansour(2012) Studies on mycosis and mycotoxicosis in cattle *Conf. of An. Health Res.*216-227.

http://www.knowmycotoxins.com/species/poultryaccessed 3/20/2019.

https://tse4.mm.bing.net/th?id=OIP.IC6jATwlp48pjFoKfUnwFQHaE6&pid=15.1&P=0&w=252 &h=168) on 12/3/2019.

https://www.cfs.gov.hk/english/programme/programme_rafs/files/cfs_news_ras_23_och.pdf accessed on 3/19/2019.

http://www.knowmycotoxins.com/species/equine accessed on 3/20/2019.

https://www.apsnet.org/edcenter/intropp/topics/Mycotoxins/Pages/EconomicImpact.aspx accessed on 13/3/2019

Iheshiulor.M.O.O.,Esonu.B.O.,Chuwuka.O.K.,Omede.A.A,Okoli.I.C.,Ogbuewu.I.P.(201 1) Effects of Mycotoxins in Animal Nutrition *Asian Journal of AnimalSciences***5** 1: 19-33

Ismaiel, A.A.; Papenbrock, J. Mycotoxins: Producing fungi and mechanisms of phytotoxicity. Agriculture 2015, 5, 492–537.

Kagot V.,OkothS.,DeBoevreM.,DeSaeger S.,(2019) Biocontrol of Aspergillus and FusariumMycotoxins in Africa: Benefits and Limitations*Toxins,***11**,109

Kaushik A.,Arya S. K., Vasudvev A., Bhansali S.(2013) Recent Advances in Detection ofOchratoxin-A *Open Journal of Applied Biosensor,***2**, 1-11

Keller L.,Abrunhosa L., Keller K. , Rosa C. A. , Cavaglieri L. and Venancio A. (2015) Zearalenone and Its Derivatives α-Zearalenol and β-Zearalenol Decontamination by Saccharomyces cerevisiae Strains Isolated from Bovine Forage *Toxins*, **7**, 3297-3308;

Kotowicz, N. K., Frac, M., and Lipiec, J. (2014). The importance of Fusarium fungi in wheat cultivation–pathogenicity and mycotoxins production: a review. *J. Anim. Plant Sci.***21**, 3326–3243

Li, Y.; Zhang, B.; He, X.; Cheng, W.H.; Xu, W.; Luo, Y.; Liang, R.; Luo, H.; Huang,(2014) K. Analysis of individual and combined effects of ochratoxin A and zearalenone on HepG2 and KK-1 cells with mathematical models. *Toxins*, 6, 1177–1192.

Lon W. W. and Winston M. Hagler, Jr. (2005)Mycotoxins in Dairy Cattle: Occurrence, Toxicity, Prevention and Treatment. *Proc. Southwest Nutr.Conf* 124-138

Milicevic, D., Juric, V., Stefanovic, S., Jovanovic, M., Jankovic, S., 2008.Survey of slaughtered pigs for occurrence of ochratoxin A and porcine nephropathy in Serbia.*Int. J. Mol. Sci.* 9, 2169– 2183

Mobashar M., Hummel J., Blank R., Südekum K.H.(2010) Ochratoxin A in Ruminants–A Review on Its Degradation by Gut Microbes and Effects on Animals *Toxins*, **2**, 809-839; doi:10.3390/toxins2040809

Mohd-Redzwan, S., Jamaluddin, R., Mutalib, A., Sokhini, M., and Ahmad, Z. (2013). A mini review on aflatoxin exposure in Malaysia: past, present and future. *Front. Microbiol.*4:334. doi: 10.3389/fmicb.2013.00334

NeleeshT:(http://www.biologydiscussion.com/fungi/classification-of-mycotoxins-fungi/46696) accessed on 19/3/2019

Peterson, S.W., Ito, Y., Horn, B.W., Goto, T., (2001).Aspergillusbombycis, a new aflatoxigenic species and genetic variation in its sibling species, A. nomius.*Mycologia,* **93**, 689–703

Rad u l o v i cJ .Z. P.,Dosen R. D. D., Stoj a n o v I.M., Pusic I. M., Balos M. M.Z., Ratajac R .D., KapetanovM. S.(2013) Influence of mycotoxinzearalenone on the swine reproductive failure. **124**, 121—129

Raju M., Devegowda G.(2000) Influence of esterified-glucomannan on performance and organ morphology, serum biochemistry and haematology in broilers exposed to individual and combined mycotoxicosis (aflatoxin, ochratoxin and T-2 toxin) *Brit. Poult. Sci.* ;**41**:640–650

Ren, G.X.; Hu, Y.C.; Zhang, J.M.; Zou, L.; Zhao, G.(2018) Determination of multi-class mycotoxins in tartary buckwheat by ultra-fast liquid chromatography coupled with triple quadrupole mass spectrometry. *Toxins,* **10**

Reyes M. https://www.poultryworld.net/Nutrition/Partner/2017/8/Mycotoxins-A-major-worry-for-organic-poultry-171071E/ accessed on 3/20/19.

Schwarzer, K., 2009. Harmful effects of mycotoxins on animal physiology. In: 17th Annual ASAIM SEA Feed Technology and Nutrition Workshop, Hue, Vietnam

Suttajit M.(http://www.fao.org/3/X5036E/x5036E0q.htm) accepted from website on 14/3/2019.

Van Egmond, H.P. (Ed.), Mycotoxins in Dairy Products. Elsevier Applied Science, London, pp. 11–55.

Zain Mohamed E. (2011) Impact of mycotoxins on humans and animals *Journal of Saudi Chemical Society*, **15**, 129–144.

Zheng W., Wang B.,, Xi Li.,Wang T.,Zou H.,JianhongGuJ.,YuanY., Liu X.,Bai J.,Bian J., Liu z.(2010) Zearalenone Promotes Cell Proliferation or Causes Cell Death?*Toxins,***10**, 184 1-17.

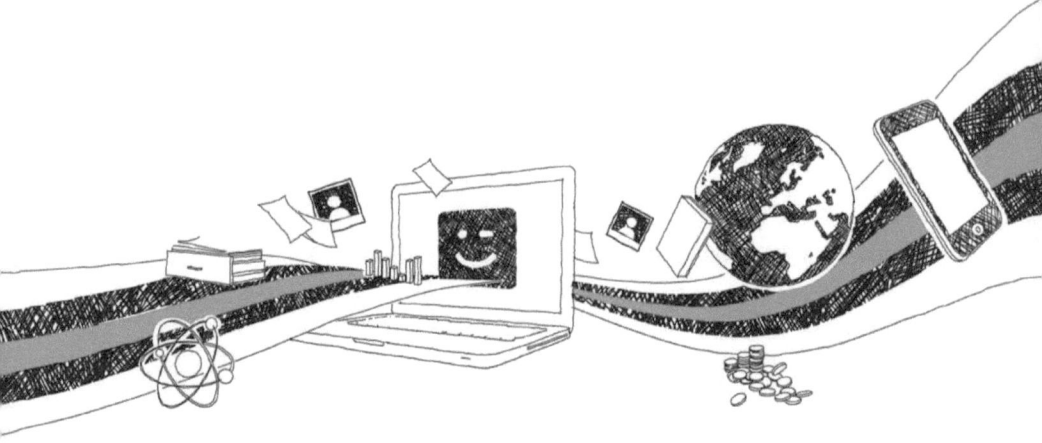
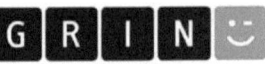